Relaxation For Breastfeeding!

A Guidebook Journal

Insert photo here

Anita McGruder-Johnson, PhD
and Vernell Johnson III, MD

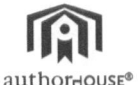

authorHOUSE®

AuthorHouse™
1663 Liberty Drive, Suite 200
Bloomington, IN 47403
www.authorhouse.com
Phone: 1-800-839-8640

First published by AuthorHouse 3/18/2010

ISBN: 978-1-4343-3406-0 (sc)

Library of Congress Control Number: 2007906179

Printed in the United States of America
Bloomington, Indiana

This book is printed on acid-free paper.

TABLE OF CONTENTS

Dear Mommy,

Congratulations! Breastfeeding is a great choice for newborn nourishment. When I had my children, I knew that I wanted to breastfeed each one. I talked to other mothers and read a lot of materials.

I learned that healthy lactation has been associated with four components: relaxation, breast emptying, nutrition and hydration. When I combined these elements, I found that I was more capable of producing milk for my baby.

I felt more relaxed and able to enjoy the time with my infant. A nurse also told me while I was in the hospital, that if I really tried for 2 weeks, I would learn to breastfeed my baby and become comfortably competent.

I shared these tips with my sister-in-law and a friend who had a pre-term infant, and they reported similar results. I hope these ideas help you as they have helped me.

Best to you,
Anita McGruder-Johnson, PhD

Author's Note

This book is meant to complement, not substitute for, the advice given by your physician. The authors have exerted effort to provide the most current information, however in light of ongoing research in this field it is possible that new findings may invalidate some of the data presented here.

Agencies, authors, organizations and websites mentioned in this book are included for informational purposes and do not indicate affiliation.

According to the Center for Disease Control, HIV may be transmitted in breastmilk. It is recommended that women who are HIV+ should not breastfeed. Further discussion of these and other related issues are available on the website [www.ashastd.org/nah/].

FOREWORD

It was the forty-second week of my first pregnancy and I was completely exhausted. All I could think about was having this baby so I could get some sleep! Although this seemed naive, it was no understatement; this view is shared by many other pregnant mothers.

After the delivery, I was joyous, fatigued, and sore. All I could now envision was nurturing my baby. It is well known that breastfeeding is a very healthy decision for baby well-being. I knew that women had been breastfeeding for centuries. Yet, I was struggling and my breasts were sore. "Latching on" was a challenge, and my letdown was slow because of fatigue. I even read somewhere that some tribal communities shared breastfeeding duty among several lactating mothers. However, like me, many nursing mothers are "flying solo" every day and every night.

A lactation specialist told me that stress was reducing my milk supply and that relaxation was all I needed. How can a breastfeeding mother relax when the stress comes from trying to breastfeed? After reading, relaxing, meditating, experiencing, and enduring many trials, breastfeeding became a very natural process.

Milk production is also a natural scientific process. It is learned, practiced, modified, and practiced more. Your body adjusts. The baby adjusts. The milk is established and maintained for healthy nutrition, and all is well with the world.

We embarked on this project to provide practical information about the training process of breastfeeding. When you choose to breastfeed, you are also choosing to commit time and effort to acquiring a new skill.

Our intention is to share what we have learned as a breastfeeding couple. In addition to practical information, we will present some of the research literature examining the underlying biological and psychological mechanisms that influence milk supply. In particular, we will examine the links between relaxation and lactation.

This *Guidebook Journal*™ is a resource for the *Relaxation for Breastfeeding and Skin-to-Skin Infant Care!* audio that will lead you through positioning, breathing, relaxing, visualizing, meditating, and affirming exercises.

CHAPTER 1

Preparing To Make Milk

Mindfulness and Maternity: Mommies Need Relaxation

Relaxation for Breastfeeding supports a holistic approach to nursing support. It is based on experiences of breastfeeding mothers as well as biology, and psychology.

Lactogenesis is the process of milk production.[1] This process is influenced by the mind and the body. You provide the hormones following the delivery of a newborn. If the nipples are stimulated during this period, you should make milk.[2,3] Nipples are stimulated by the suckling baby or a breast pump. Such stimulation influences the release of oxytocin, a hormone that signals the letdown of milk.[1,4,5]

The contented mommy produces the best milk! To be content, you have to relax. Relaxation and imagery techniques have been used to help mothers with spinal cord injuries above the breasts produce milk for their newborns.[5]

If paralyzed mothers can enhance their milk production by relaxing, then it is worth a try. Relaxation influences the release of oxytocin, but experiencing stress and secreting adrenalin may block its release.[6-9] In fact, lactating mothers may be especially good at relaxing because maternal hormones (e.g., oxytocin and prolactin) promote calmness – an effect that can last after nursing has ceased. Essentially, you may be able to achieve a deeper state of relaxation now and in the future because you have practiced in the presence of your natural sedative—oxytocin.

When you feel pressured or overwhelmed, you are experiencing stress. It accompanies all life events—good events as well as bad events. The body responds to this pressure by breaking down.[9,10]

Taking care of a newborn can be very stressful. During the time when a mother requires rest and relaxation, the sleep schedule is controlled by the newborn. Lack of sleep and frequent demands from a newborn, significant others, siblings, or a job can overwhelm a mother.

Since each child is different, the postnatal adjustment period can be full of stressors; even the seasoned mommy will feel stressed. Some people blame it on hormones, but the numerous demands of motherhood, relationships and daily living can affect the emotions as well.

Moms often find that they experience a range of emotions. Sometimes moms experience "postpartum blues" or even severe symptoms of depression.[4] Therefore, the postnatal period is an important time for a mother to take some moments to relax and rejuvenate. You may find that when you allow yourself some moments to relax, thoughts that worry you become less intense.

Whether you are nursing or expressing your milk, relaxation can be beneficial. Make relaxation a part of your breastfeeding routine. Try it for fourteen consecutive days. If you choose, you may want to consider your level of tension before and after the relaxation period.

Using a rating scale of one (Very Relaxed) to seven (Very Tense), allow the number to come into your mind that best describes how you are feeling and write it in your journal (see Appendix A). Remember: do this again after your relaxation session. Additionally, write down the positive (pleasant, nice, comforting) thoughts and feelings that you experienced during the session.

Mommies Need Self-Care

Women have frequently assisted each other during the maternity, childbirth, and postpartum periods. Unfortunately, the structure of contemporary society has limited this benefit for contemporary breastfeeding women. This section consists of suggestions to enhance this experience for you. For additional information, contact La Leche League International, a not-for-profit organization that promotes breastfeeding by providing resources to the public (see Appendix B).

- Before nursing (or pumping), prepare the breasts by taking a warm shower or bath or by placing a moist, warm (not hot) towel upon the breasts.

- Always break the suction before removing the baby from your nipple. Place your index finger gently inside the edge of the baby's mouth closest to your breastbone and release the suction to prevent damage to your skin.

- If you have discomfort during or following breastfeeding, consider a lanolin product manufactured for soothing the nipples.

- Lactation requires rest. Sleep when the baby sleeps! This is the best advice for moms of newborns. When your baby is bigger, you may be able to do housekeeping and other chores while carrying the infant in a baby carrier.

- Eat a healthy snack during or following each nursing or expression session. Drink plenty of fluids throughout the day and night.

- To increase your milk production, *empty your breast*. Pump or nurse every two to three hours for at least twenty minutes. If you pump simultaneously while nursing, your body may think you are feeding twins and increase the amount of milk that it produces (i.e., supply and demand).

  o Sample schedule:

  5:00 a.m., 8:00 a.m., 11:00 a.m., 2:00 p.m., 5:00 p.m., 8:00 p.m., 11:00 p.m., 2:00 a.m..

- Keep a journal of your thoughts about this time in your life.

- Know that other women have had some of the experiences that you are having now. Consider attending activities for moms and tots.

- Take a mental health break.

- Do not be afraid to ask for help!

- Ask for specific help (e.g., have friends or family who want to give you a gift prepare dinner meals for a week).

Spouse Spotlight On Relaxation And Self-Care

- Spouses can bottle feed expressed milk day or night.

- Around-the-clock infant care can be rough for all.

  Keep yourself calm. Monitor your stress level.

- You can ask for help too.

- Give soothing touches.

- Shower together.

- Massage each other.

CHAPTER 2

Preparing For Skin-to-Skin Infant Care

Holding

Infants benefit from the physical comfort they receive through holding. The beauty of holding an infant is that it enhances human bonding. Mothers, fathers, grandparents, adoptive parents and other caregivers can share the gift of physical comfort with an infant. When you are relaxed, the comfort increases. The "...Skin-to-Skin..." track on the *Breastfeeding for Relaxation and Skin-To-Skin Infant Care!* audio CD can be used as an accompaniment during these precious moments.

This section presents information about skin-to-skin snuggling (a.k.a., "kangaroo care") – holding your diapered infant (with its head upright) against the skin of your chest while gently supporting its body in your arms. Sitting in a recliner may provide the most comfort and support of your head neck and back while snuggling your baby. Lightly cover the infant's body (not its face) with your shirt or a baby blanket.

Bonding

You may notice that your baby cuddles against your warmth, breathing in your scent while feeling your heart's familiar cadence guiding each breath in and out. This is a natural connection between you and your baby, resembling the safety and comfort of the womb. Such skin-to-skin infant cuddling can strengthen emotional connectedness and mental health.[16,17,18] Your baby learns that it can rely on you for safety, comfort and relaxation; and this sense of security and comfort helps your baby to thrive.

Since the beginning of time, infants have been cuddled closely to their caregivers. In fact, research indicates that skin-to-skin contact with the chest of a <u>female</u> or <u>male</u> can help to control the infant's breathing and body temperature.[19,20,21] If the caregiver helps to control breathing and body warmth, cuddled infants can use more of their energy towards growth and development, rather than survival itself.

Caring

Skin-to-skin snuggling can enhance the care you give during these early days, weeks, months, during weaning, and throughout the early toddler years. Each beat of your heart guides the continued development of your baby's brain during soothing rest and sleep. Each beat of your heart reminds you that caring for your baby can be peaceful and healthy. It is so nice that a simple cuddle can create amazing benefits to your child. As your baby gets older, the two of you will continue to adjust to each other in a way that optimizes development, health and security.

Make relaxation a part of your skin-to-skin snuggling routine. You may want to consider your level of tension before and after the relaxation snuggling period. Using a rating scale of one (Very Relaxed) to seven (Very Tense), allow the number to come into your mind that best describes how you are feeling and write it in your journal (see Appendix A). Remember: do this again after your relaxation session. Additionally, write down the positive (pleasant, nice, comforting) thoughts and feelings that you experienced during the session.

Spouse Spotlight on Skin-to-Skin Infant Care and Bonding

- Skin-to-skin infant snuggling is a great way to bond with your baby.
- Snuggle while reading, feeding and relaxing.
- Consider "wearing" the baby during daily activities or light exercise (using an approved infant wearing device).
- Give yourself permission to enjoy comfort and peace from a skin-to-skin snuggle.
- Snuggle with mommy skin-to-skin, too!

CHAPTER 3

Preparing For Stressors

Planning

Every day in life, we experience changes that produce varying degrees of emotional distress (sadness, anger, fright, frustration). In order to enhance our health and parenting, we must manage our stress.

- Identify the stressors (i.e., the issues that make you feel sad, angry, scared or frustrated).
- Make a stress-management plan.
- Use the plan.

Your stress-management plan may be as simple as taking slow, deep breaths. When you become distressed (sad, angry, scared, frustrated), your heart rate and breathing speed up. If you can force them to become slower at these times, you may improve your health and give yourself time to respond—not react.

Positioning

You don't have to sit in the dark, but you can do things that can help you achieve a more relaxed state. You can recline with your head, neck, and back supported while elevating your legs.

Place the infant on a pillow in your lap (with the infant's head facing the ceiling) so that the baby's body is fully supported by the pillow in case you fall asleep. Be sure that nothing covers the baby's face. A recliner may provide the best support for you and the infant.

Breathing

Close your eyes and get ready to start relaxing (e.g., uncross you arms and legs). Begin by taking slow, deep breaths.

One of the most important parts of relaxation is breathing. You want to inhale slowly through your nostrils, forcing your stomach to push forward. This is different from the way we usually breathe, but it will allow your lungs to obtain more air.

Exhale through your mouth on a count of three. If you find that you are struggling as though you are holding your breath, you may want to use a count of two.

Practice this type of breathing until you can feel yourself relaxing. You may find that the more you practice, the faster you will become relaxed. After you establish your breathing, you may want to enhance your experience via guided relaxation, visualization, and meditation techniques included on the audio portion of this lactation support system.

Relaxing

When you experience relaxation, your body is able to produce milk. As you become more relaxed, you may notice warm or tingling sensations in your breasts. It may start at the sides of your breasts and flow downward toward the nipples. There may be some slight discomfort, but it will not bother you much, because you will know it means that you are making milk for your baby and that the milk is coming down toward your nipples.

How exciting it is to be able to give life to and nourishment to an infant! You may want to help the process by allowing pleasant thoughts to surround your mind. Mothering does not need perfection. This is a special experience that comes from your love for your baby, and any amount of milk you can make for your baby will be beneficial. In fact, babies receive their ability to fight infection from the colostrum in their mothers' milk![4]

Visualizing

Allowing an image, color, or word to come into your mind can help you feel more relaxed, more content, and more comfortable. The image should symbolize peace, calmness, and contentment. For example, try to envision a warm sun shining brightly in the sky. Paint it vividly in your mind so that you can experience its warmth.

Sometimes imagining the warmth of wet water can increase your relaxation. Let the warm liquid surround and soothe your body. Feel the sensations as they travel on your skin. Allow yourself to welcome a more relaxed state of being.

Meditating and Affirming

Meditation can be used with or without relaxation. You may find that reading or reciting an affirmative statement helps you to feel less tense. There are original poems written below.

Some of the sentiments may fit you better than others. Allow the words that are meaningful to your situation to resonate. If you become inspired, you may choose to write about it in your journal or use some of your own experiences when you meditate.

Smile

When I see my infants smile, it makes me smile.

As my baby looks into my eyes, I am filled with awe.

This baby is too special to describe.

I want to be the protector and provide nourishment

that supports the growth of my child.

Meaning of Tears

My child . . . wow . . .

Sometimes I am filled with so many emotions I just cry.

The tears have many meanings.

I cry for happiness, for fears, for love, for responsibility, for hope, for

the future.

I am amazed every day by my baby's sheer existence.

I Am Enough

I am sometimes tired, overwhelmed, and concerned that I cannot be

everything to my child or mold a healthy, well-adjusted person.

But today, for this moment, I am enough.

I Will Learn

Sometimes I do not know how to comfort my child.

When the cries come at night and I am asleep,

When I think all of the needs are met and my baby wants to be

held . . .

I am willing to learn with my child.

Baby Language

I want to know my infant's ways of communication:

The language of cries, coos, and gurgles,

The language of reaches, starts, and kicks,

The way my child lets me know what to do and when to do it.

Above all, I want to know the language that tells me I can be the

mother my baby needs, and I can care for myself that way too!

One Moment, One Step

It seems like there are so many things to do now; I do not know

where to begin.

The day starts and I am already behind schedule.

My energy seems to run out after doing fewer tasks.

How do I recapture my life when things are so different now?

I take one moment and one step at a time.

Emotions

Sometimes the responsibility overwhelms me. My emotions are

turbulent:

I laugh, I cry, I hope, I fear, I wish.

So now I take my moments to breathe;

I breathe in peace and breathe out confusion.

Spouse Spotlight On Intimacy And Stress Management

- Enjoy relaxing together. Cradle Mommy as she cradles your baby.

- Switch places: Mommy cradles you while you give kangaroo care (skin-to-skin infant care).

- Reflect together on positive feelings experienced during this special time.

CHAPTER 4

Preparing Healthier Meals

Healthier Food Choices

Breastfeeding can stimulate your appetite. Although you are eating for two, you need only consume five hundred extra calories per day.[11] This is not the time to binge on high fat, high sugar foods, nor is it the time to engage in strict weight-reduction dieting.

The calories required by an infant are taken from the milk it consumes. These calories come from the mom. The baby gets out of the milk what is put into it. So it is important to make healthier food choices.

Many Mini Meals

Try eating a small snack and drinking eight to sixteen ounces of water, juice or noncaffeinated tea during or after nursing or the expressing of your milk. Consider keeping a crate of bottled water and a basket of healthy goodies nearby (in the nursery, beside your bed, or in other places where you tend to nurse you baby).

The Goody Basket	The Refrigerator
fruit cups	yogurt
oatmeal cookies	fresh fruit
bottles of water	low-fat turkey meat
bottles of juice	cheese slices

For meals, select foods from each of the food groups: fruits, vegetables, whole grains, low-fat milk and milk products, and lean proteins. Limit foods high in cholesterol, sodium, or added sugars.[12] Avoid foods high in fat (e.g., saturated fats, trans fats) or foods that may produce gas or bloating. Avoid foods that may cause allergic reactions or illness, such as peanuts, shellfish, undercooked or raw meats, and cheeses.

Herbal Assistants

Certain herbs (called herbal galactagogues) have been associated with enhancing lactation.[3,4,13,14] Common methods of ingesting herbs include tinctures, capsules, and teas. Although it is common practice, the research literature is sparse regarding this issue.

It is unclear whether the observed lactogenic effects are directly or indirectly caused by the herbs.[3,4,13,14] For instance, fenugreek is an herb that is used in lactation teas and is considered safe.[13] However, drinking fenugreek or other herbs in tea may indirectly promote milk production by increasing the volume of liquid intake (i.e., increasing hydration).[14]

Further, simply believing that herbs are increasing milk supply may lead to an increase. This is called a placebo effect.[4]

Promotion of relaxation may be another indirect lactogenic effect of herbs. Fennel seed is an herb that has been used throughout the ages for its flavor as well as its lactogenic and soothing properties.[4,14] According to the *Physician's Desk Reference of Herbal Medicines*,[15] fennel seed may also ease digestion by muscle spasm reduction (an antispasmodic effect). Ease of digestion is a sign of enhanced relaxation.

For a detailed exploration of herbs used by nursing mothers, read *The Nursing Mother's Herbal* by Sheila Humphrey.[13] Before trying herbs, consult a board-certified lactation consultant. You can find one through La Leche League International (www.LLLI.org). In addition, notify your physician to determine if using herbal galactogogues is safe for you. You may find that breast emptying, relaxation, hydration, and healthy eating are enough to help you make milk for your baby.

More Oatmeal Cookies, Please

Oatmeal can be beneficial to a lactating mom. Oats lower cholesterol and improve heart health, and they have been used to improve the milk production of dairy animals.[13]

You can eat slow-cooked oatmeal as hot cereal, but why not eat oatmeal cookies! Make a big batch of oatmeal cookies to keep on hand for snacks at home and away from home. They fit nicely in a diaper bag, snack basket or breast pump case.

More Liquids and Vitamins

Consume liquids to prevent thirst. When you experience thirst, you may be slightly dehydrated.[4] Vegetable soup is an excellent choice for nutrition and hydration. It contains few calories and lots of vitamins. The liquid from the soup helps to replenish your body's store of water.

Continue to take your prenatal vitamins! You can also drink low-sodium vegetable juices. This is a great way to increase your vegetable intake while increasing your hydration. At least two to four servings of fruits and three to four servings of vegetables are recommended by the American Academy of Pediatrics.[4]

Spouse Spotlight on Healthier Eating

- Healthy snacking is for spouses, too!
- Enjoy snacks together.
- If you maintain your health, you will find it easier to manage stress.
- Help to keep a good supply of healthy foods in the pantry.
- Bake cookies together.

Appendix A

Fourteen-Day Relaxation Journal

Relaxation Journal
Day 1

Before:

1	2	3	4	5	6	7
very relaxed			medium			very tense

After:

1	2	3	4	5	6	7
very relaxed			medium			very tense

Reflection:

Relaxation Journal
Day 2

Before:

1	2	3	4	5	6	7
very relaxed			medium			very tense

After:

1	2	3	4	5	6	7
very relaxed			medium			very tense

Reflection:

Relaxation Journal
Day 3

Before:

1	2	3	4	5	6	7
very			medium			very
relaxed						tense

After:

1	2	3	4	5	6	7
very			medium			very
relaxed						tense

Reflection:

Relaxation Journal
Day 4

Before:

1	2	3	4	5	6	7
very			medium			very
relaxed						tense

After:

1	2	3	4	5	6	7
very			medium			very
relaxed						tense

Reflection:

Relaxation Journal
Day 5

Before:

1	2	3	4	5	6	7
very relaxed			medium			very tense

After:

1	2	3	4	5	6	7
very relaxed			medium			very tense

Reflection:

Relaxation Journal
Day 6

Before:

1	2	3	4	5	6	7
very relaxed			medium			very tense

After:

1	2	3	4	5	6	7
very relaxed			medium			very tense

Reflection:

Relaxation Journal
Day 7

Before:

1	2	3	4	5	6	7
very relaxed			medium			very tense

After:

1	2	3	4	5	6	7
very relaxed			medium			very tense

Reflection:

Relaxation Journal
Day 8

Before:

1	2	3	4	5	6	7
very relaxed			medium			very tense

After:

1	2	3	4	5	6	7
very relaxed			medium			very tense

Reflection:

Relaxation Journal
Day 9

Before:

1	2	3	4	5	6	7
very relaxed			medium			very tense

After:

1	2	3	4	5	6	7
very relaxed			medium			very tense

Reflection:

Relaxation Journal
Day 10

Before:

1	2	3	4	5	6	7
very relaxed			medium			very tense

After:

1	2	3	4	5	6	7
very relaxed			medium			very tense

Reflection:

Relaxation Journal
Day 11

Before:

1	2	3	4	5	6	7
very			medium			very
relaxed						tense

After:

1	2	3	4	5	6	7
very			medium			very
relaxed						tense

Reflection:

Relaxation Journal
Day 12

Before:

1	2	3	4	5	6	7
very			medium			very
relaxed						tense

After:

1	2	3	4	5	6	7
very			medium			very
relaxed						tense

Reflection:

Relaxation Journal
Day 13

Before:

1	2	3	4	5	6	7
very			medium			very
relaxed						tense

After:

1	2	3	4	5	6	7
very			medium			very
relaxed						tense

Reflection:

Relaxation Journal
Day 14

Before:

1	2	3	4	5	6	7
very relaxed			medium			very tense

After:

1	2	3	4	5	6	7
very relaxed			medium			very tense

Reflection:

APPENDIX B

Resources and References

Resources for Caregivers

In this section, we have listed websites and contact information for organizations, support groups, and hotlines that provide resources for parents of small children.
In particular, we have included breastfeeding, abuse, HIV/AIDS, poison control, and other medical and mental health resources. In an emergency, call 911 where available.

- American Academy of Pediatrics [www.aap.org]

- Center for Disease Control National AIDS Hotline [1-800-342-AIDS]

- Center for Disease Control National STD Hotline [1-800-227-8922 English 1-800-344-7432 Spanish]

- Healthy Sensations International [www.naturalhealthsensations.com]

- Healthy Sensations Greatest Relaxation Hits! [www.cdbaby.com/all/relax]

- La Leche League International [www.lalecheleague.org]

- March of Dimes [www.modimes.org]

- Mocha Moms [www.mochamoms.org]

- Mothers of Preschoolers (MOPS) [www. mothersofpresechoolers.com]

- National Child Abuse Hotline [1-800-4ACHILD]

- National Domestic Violence Hotline [1-800-799- SAFE (7233) or

  1-800-787-3224 (TDD)]

- National Hope Line Network [1-800 SUICIDE or 1-800-784-2433]

- National Women's Health Information Center U.S. Department of Health and Human Services [www.4women.gov/breastfeeding /AABA]

- Parents Anonymous [www.parentsanonymous.org]

- Planned Parenthood Federation of America [www. plannedparenthood.org]

- Poison Control [1-800-222-1222]

- United States Department of Agriculture (USDA) [www.MyPyramid.gov]

- U. S. Product Safety Commission [www.cpsc.gov] (800) 637- 2772 (consumer hotline)

References

1. Riordan, J. *Breastfeeding and Human Lactation*. 3rd ed.. Sudbury, Mass: Jones and Bartlett Publishers, 2005.

2. Groh-Wargo, S., A. Toth, K. Mahoney, S. Simonian, T. Wasser, and S. Rose. The utility of a bilateral breast pumping system for mothers of premature infants. *Neonatal Network* 14 (1995): 31–36.

3. Mohrbacher, N. and J. Stock. *The Breastfeeding Answer Book*. 3rd ed. Schamburg, Illinois: La Leche League International, 2002.

4. American Academy of Pediatrics (AAP). *New mother's guide to breastfeeding*. New York: Bantam Books, 2002.

5. Cowley, K. C. "Psychogenic and Pharmacologic Induction of the Let-down Reflex Can Facilitate Breastfeeding by Tetraplegic Women: A Report of 3 Cases." *Archives of Physical Medicine and Rehabilitation* 86 no.6 (2005): 1261–4.

6. Dermer, A. "A Well-kept Secret: Breastfeeding's Benefits to Mothers." Chap. 8 in *Breastfeeding annual international 2001*. Edited by D. L. Michels. Washington, DC: Platypus Media LLC, 2001.

7. Feher, S. D., L. R. Berger, J. D. Johnson, and J. B. Wilde. "Increasing Breast Milk Production for Premature Infants

with a Relaxation/Imagery Audiotape. *Pediatrics* 83 (1989):, 57–60.

8. O'Conner, M. E., W. Schmidt, C. Carroll-Pankhurst, and K. N. Olness. "Relaxation Training and Breast Milk Secretory IgA." *Archives of pediatric and adolescent medicine* 152 (1998): 1065–1070.

9. Ueda, T., Y. Yokoyama, M. Irahara, and T. Aono. Influence of Psychological Stress on Suckling-induced Pulsatile Oxytocin Release." *Obstetrics and gynecology* 84 (1994): 259–262.

10. Manber, R., J. J. Allen, and M. M. Morris. "Alternative Treatments for Depression: Empirical Support and Relevance to Women." *Journal of Clinical Psychiatry* 63 (2002): 628–640.

11. Wright, K. S., T.J. Quinn, and G. B. Carey. "Infant Acceptance of Breast Milk After Maternal Exercise." *Pediatrics* 109 (2002): 109 585–589.

12. United States Department of Agriculture. "Dietary guidelines." http://www.mypyramid.gov/guidelines/index.html. (Accessed June 20, 2006).

13. Humphrey, S. *The Nursing Mother's Herbal*. Minneapolis, Minnesota: Fairview Press, 2003.

14. Martin, C. *The Nursing Mother's Problem Solver*. New York: Fireside, 2000.

15. Physician's Desk Reference. *PDR for herbal medicines*. Montvale, NJ: Thomson Healthcare, 2004.

16. Bowlby, J. (1969). *Attachment, Attachment and Loss*. Vol. I. London: Hogarth.

17. Bretherton, I. (1992). The origins of attachment theory: John Bowlby and Mary Ainsworth. *Developmental Psychology*, 28, 759-775.

18. Feldman, R., Weller, A., Sirota, L. and Eidelman, A. (2003). Testing a family intervention hypothesis: The contribution of mother-infant skin-to-skin contact (kangaroo care) to family interaction, proximity, and touch. *Journal of Family Psychology*, 17(1), 94-107.

19. Erlandsson, K., Dsilna, A., Faferberg, I. and Christensson, K. (2007). Skin-to-skin care with the father after cesarean birth and its effect on newborn crying and prefeeding behavior. *Birth: Issues in perinatal care*, 34(2), 105-114.

20. Ludington-Hoe, S. & Hosseini, R. (2005). Skin-to-Skin Contact Analgesia for Preterm Infant Heel Stick. *AACN Clin Issues*; 16(3): 373–387.

21. Dombrowski, M. A. S., Anderson, G. C., Santori, C., Roller, C. G., Pagliotti, F., Dowling, D. A. (2000). Kangaroo skin-to-skin care for premature twins and their adolescent parents. *The American Journal of Maternal/Child Nursing,* 25(2), 92-94.

ITEM	DESCRIPTION		#	PRICE
HOLIDAY SLEEPTIME STORIES	**Holiday Sleeptime Stories** Relaxing holiday melodies and stories, including the Nativity, Christmas, Chanukah & Kwaanza.	15.99		
	Relief of Relaxation Smooth jazz accompanying calming spoken word guides you through brief exercises to enhance stress and anger management.	15.99		
	Relaxation for Breastfeeding and Skin-To-Skin Infant Care! Calming spoken word over soft music. Guided relaxation, imagery and meditations to enhance the bonding experience.	15.99		
	SLEEPBOOST'R Guided Relaxation Story The "SLEEPBOOST'R Guided Relaxation Story CD" is to train young children to relax and prepare to resting	15.99		
	SHIPPING & HANDLING Continental United States	$15.00		
TOTAL				

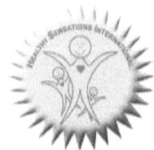

HEALTHY SENSATIONS INTERNATIONAL
WELLNESS SOLUTIONS
HEALTHIER BODIES = FULLER LIVES

Credit Card Orders:

(__)VISA   (__)MasterCard

Card holder name (as printed on card) *please print

_____

Card number __ __ __ __ - __ __ __ __ - __ __ __ __ - __ __ __ __

Expiration Date: Month:_____ Year:_____

last 3-digits on back of credit card __ __ __

I authorize Healthy Sensations International to charge

$_____ on _____ .

      invoice total   *Date*

_____
Cardholder Signature

_____
Date

Billing address (please print):

Name:_____

Address:_____

_____

E-mail: _____

Tel: (_____)-(_____)-(_____)

Fax: (_____)-(_____)-(_____)

Shipping address (please print):

Name:_____

Address:_____

_____

E-mail: _____

Tel: (_____)-(_____)-(_____)

Fax: (_____)-(_____)-(_____)

ORDER FORM/RECEIPT

FAX TO: *(708) 679-0911*   *OR*
EMAIL TO:
HSI@NATURALHEALTHSENSATIONS.COM

BOOK PREVIEW

Seven days changed the world: Seven days can change your life!

Live the life God intended: with peace, optimism, control, harmony, appreciation and rest. The Creation story provides a guide for managing big challenges. There are seven tasks. Learning and practicing these tasks will help you experience peace, joy and harmony in your daily life.

A stress-free life is available to all. Growing in peace, harmony and self-respect is a gift at any age.

INTRODUCTION--LIVING A STRESS-FREE LIFE

"I will lift up my eyes to the hills -- From where will my help come? My help comes from the Lord, who made heaven and earth."

Psalm 121:1-2

God is the ultimate role model for coping with chaos in a stress-free way. The Creation story reveals God's stress defense tasks. The world and all that dwells within it was not created in one day. God expected to be able to complete the project in an appropriate manner, despite the original chaos and disorder (Genesis 1:2). He started at the top: Light was ordered to bring clarity to the project (Genesis 1:3). One bit of the project was tackled at a time, and at the end of each day, God reflected on his work, stating "it is good" (Genesis 1: 9-31).

When man was alone in the Garden of Eden, God reconsidered the effect of loneliness and isolation on the man's ability to experience happiness in life. God created a companion, encouraging mutual support and productivity (Genesis 2:18-22). And on the seventh day, God rested (Genesis 2:2). God took care of himself, allowing for recuperation and rejuvenation in readiness to handle the next challenges.

The Creation story provides a guide for managing big challenges. There are seven tasks. Learning and practicing these tasks will help you experience peace, joy and harmony in your daily life. A stress-free life is available to all. Growing in peace, harmony and self-respect is a gift at any age.

HOW TO USE THIS

GUIDEBOOK JOURNAL

Live the life God intended: with peace, optimism, control, harmony, appreciation and rest. *7 Days To A Stress-Free Life!* teaches you how to experience more satisfaction and less stress by integrating God's stress defense tasks into your daily routine. Seek peace, break off smaller bits, expect positive outcomes, encourage yourself often, seek supportive companionship, reflect on the positive and immerse in appreciation. As you go through each day, use this guidebook journal to write about your journey from confusion to clarity, peace, and control. Each day consider your happiness and rate it on a scale from 0 (not at all happy) to 10 (very happy) and list 2 simple pleasures you experienced.

DAY ONE: SEEK PEACE

"The earth was without form, and void; and darkness was on the face of the deep. And the Spirit of God was hovering over the face of the waters."

Genesis 1:2, New King James Version

The Spirit of God is with you in the darkness hovering peacefully, reminding you that you were created in his image by his breath. A slow, purposeful breath produces a miraculous change in the body. Breath is life. God shared his breath and gave the gift of life (Genesis 2:7). This powerful gift from God is within each of us. It can help us find peace in the midst of chaos.

When we experience chaos in our thoughts, our bodies respond chaotically. Frequent worry creates a physical stress response. Stress hormones surge and the heart beats faster. The worry makes us feel overwhelmed and out of control. When this process is in full force, it's often difficult to know where to start in order to improve the situation.

When we control our breathing, we add control to our bodies. A slow, deep breath starts the path to mental clarity, emotional wellbeing and behavioral control. As you initiate each task each day, invoke the slow, healing breath given to you by God.

DAY TWO: BREAK OFF SMALLER BITS OF CONFUSION

God took on a challenge to create a world. To make order out of chaos, God split this challenge into smaller, manageable pieces. God started by giving light and awareness to the situation.

"Then God said, 'Let there be light'; and there was light."

Genesis 1:3

We will experience challenges that produce confusion. We will not experience more than we can handle. Life occurs one moment at a time in order to give us ample opportunity to find strategies to receive "light" and awareness to relieve life's confusion.

God has given you strength. Be encouraged that you have the ability to breathe in clarity to break the problem into smaller pieces and select one bit to manage during the week. Stay in peace as you write about the process.

As you break off the bit to chew on for the week, activate the specific strengths (e.g., skills, resources, character traits, equipment) that will help you manage the issue. Our strengths are revealed in our sources of joy. For example, I enjoy reading mysteries. As the story unfolds, the suspense builds. I don't skip ahead, but read each word, each sentence and each page until I uncover the mystery. This process requires patience. I become aware that "Patience" is one of my strengths. Patience will help me manage bits of confusion this week.

DAY THREE: EXPECT POSITIVE OUTCOMES

God never doubted that a world could be created by just speaking it into existence. These expectations held the power to create new possibilities. The heavens and earth were created: mountains were moved and water was placed into oceans, rivers and seas.

Our expectations hold the power to move mountains, too. Unfortunately, negative expectations often get in the way. When we doubt, we reduce our power to create new possibilities. We stop considering new alternatives assuming we are already defeated.

What you do can make a difference. Positive outcomes include the stamina to stand through the tough moment until the calmer moment. You can be effective in improving your life. Just expect it!

DAY FOUR: ENCOURAGE YOURSELF OFTEN

"And God saw that the light was good;..."

Genesis 1:4

"God called the dry land Earth, and the water that was gathered together, he called Seas. And God saw that it was good."

Genesis 1:10

"The Earth brought forth vegetation:...
And God saw that it was good."

Genesis 1:12

God separated "...the light from the darkness.
And God saw that it was good."

Genesis 1:18

God created fish and birds. "... And God saw that it was good."

Genesis 1:21

"And God made the wild animals of the earth of every kind.... And God saw that it was good."

Genesis 1:25

"God saw everything that He had made, and indeed,

it was very good."

Genesis 1:31

"And it was good"....These simple words empowered God to continue creating. God reflected on His work and was pleased. God gives us permission to encourage our effort as often as we think about it.

What you say to yourself matters. Our thoughts create a constant chatter in our minds. As I type this book, I "hear" the words in my mind. As you go through each moment in life, your self-chatter goes with you.

What you chatter to yourself can hurt and discourage your efforts. Imagine having a conversation for several years with someone who only discourages, doubts and dissuades you from trying. Discouraging self-chatter can disrupt the flow of useful ideas that lead you to a positive path.

Be God-like as you chat to yourself. Remember: In God's eyes, it is good. If you notice you are doubting your abilities, you can cheer for yourself instead. Become your biggest fan. Send yourself encouraging thoughts, notes, emails and texts messages. You can become your greatest source of encouragement, affirmation and validation.

DAY FIVE: SEEK SUPPORTIVE COMPANIONSHIP

18   And the Lord God said, 'it is not good that man should be alone; I will make him a helper comparable to him.'

19   Out of the ground, the Lord God formed every beast of the field and every bird of the air, and brought them to Adam to see what he would call them. And whatever Adam called each creature, that was its name.

20   So Adam gave names to all cattle, to the birds of the air, and to every beast of the field. But for Adam there was not found a helper comparable to him.

21   And the Lord caused a great sleep to fall on Adam, and he slept; And he took one of his ribs, and closed up the flesh in its place.

22   Then the rib which God had taken from man He made into a woman,...

Genesis 2: 18-22, New King James Version

When man was alone in the Garden of Eden, God reconsidered the effect of loneliness and isolation on the man's ability to experience happiness in life. God considered several animals and decided something new and different was needed for this particular situation. God was innovative when God created a companion from the resources available. God sought harmony and mutual support to establish efficiency and productivity.

God created us to interact with each other in harmony. When conflict occurs, it escalates because anger and hostile reactions are triggered. The body prepares itself to fight or flee. The ignited fuse burns intensely and spreads quickly.

Conflict may arise, but it can be minimized. Remember the healing breath from DAY 1? Breathe is slowly to enhance calmness and clarity, allowing you the time to consider the consequences of different responses. With God's calming breath flowing, you will find a calmer response.

DAY SIX: REFLECT ON THE POSITIVE

"God saw everything that He had made, and indeed, it was
very good."

Genesis 1:31

Misery loves miserable company. When we are stressed, it is
easier to notice the negative. Sometimes it is easier to notice what
is going wrong and troubling you throughout the day. If we are
bombarded by negatives, we assume that is all that exists.

Focus instead on what is going well and right. Give yourself
credit for the many things you accomplish each moment. We must
reprogram ourselves to see the positive moments in our lives. God
surrounds us with simple pleasures: the smell of flowers, a cool breeze,
gently falling snowflakes, a warm cup of tea, a kind smile and soothing
melody. Spending time experiencing simple pleasures opens the
doorway toward stress-free living.

DAY SEVEN: IMMERSE IN APPRECIATION

"And on the 7th day,… [God] rested…"

Genesis 2:2

God allowed time to rest and recuperate. As your stress defense role model, God demonstrates the importance of self-appreciation and self-care. Appreciation is powerful medicine.

It reminds us of the positive connections we have with ourselves and others, generating feelings that warm our hearts and minds. Appreciation combats stress.

Appreciate yourself and your efforts by caring for yourself. Give attention to neglected parts of your body. Give soothing to aching areas – these are the parts of your body that are really trying to work for you. Give yourself a smile I the mirror. Send yourself a cheerful thought, note, email or text. Identify the high stress day of your week and give yourself a gift on that day. Use a calendar to remind yourself to appreciate positives and make healthier choices for the next 7 days.

INDEX

www.ingramcontent.com/pod-product-compliance
Lightning Source LLC
Chambersburg PA
CBHW021240280526
45784CB00005B/2178